# ARTHRITIS

# ALLEVIATION

## Modern Therapies For Joint Health And Pain Management

**Empower Yourself With The Knowledge Of Advanced Arthritis Therapies To Live A Pain-Free And Active Lifestyle**

**DR. BRIDGET PROMISE**

# Table of Contents

# CHAPTER ONE

## Introduction

Arthritis is a common and sometimes misunderstood medical illness that affects millions of individuals throughout the globe. The word "arthritis" refers to joint inflammation that causes pain, stiffness, and limited movement.

Because this disorder may have a substantial influence on an individual's quality of life, it is critical to grasp its intricacies, different forms, and typical symptoms.

In this examination, we will dig into the fundamentals of arthritis, learning about its origins, the many varieties that exist, and the symptoms that people may encounter.

## Arthritis Explained

Arthritis is fundamentally a joint illness marked by inflammation. Joints, or the connections between bones, are essential for our bodies to move. Arthritis causes pain and suffering by interfering with the regular functioning of these joints.

Arthritic inflammation may damage not just the joints but also the surrounding tissues and other connective systems.

There are about 100 different varieties of arthritis, each with its own set of characteristics, causes, and treatment options. The most frequent types are osteoarthritis and rheumatoid arthritis, each of which has distinct features and affects people differently.

The most common kind, osteoarthritis, is caused by the wear and tear of joint cartilage over time. Cartilage is the protective tissue that covers the ends of bones in a joint; when it deteriorates, bones may rub against one other, causing discomfort, swelling, and decreased flexibility. Weight-bearing joints, such as the knees, hips, and spine, are often affected by this kind of arthritis.

Rheumatoid arthritis, on the other hand, is an autoimmune illness in which the body's immune system erroneously targets the synovium, the lining of the membranes surrounding the joints. This causes inflammation, which might eventually lead to joint abnormalities. Rheumatoid arthritis, unlike osteoarthritis, may affect several joints at the same time and may also affect other organs and systems inside the body.

## The Various Types of Arthritis

Aside from osteoarthritis and rheumatoid arthritis, there are many different varieties of arthritis, each with its own set of traits and causes. Psoriatic arthritis, ankylosing spondylitis, gout, and juvenile idiopathic arthritis are a few examples.

Psoriatic arthritis is common in those who have the skin disorder psoriasis. It may affect any joint and can develop spondylitis, or inflammation of the spine. Ankylosing spondylitis typically affects the spine, producing inflammation and perhaps causing the vertebrae to fuse over time.

Gout is a kind of arthritis caused by the buildup of uric acid crystals in the joints, resulting in severe pain and inflammation. It usually affects the big toe, although it may also affect other joints. Juvenile idiopathic arthritis refers to a group of arthritis forms that afflict youngsters and cause joint pain, swelling, and stiffness.

These many forms of arthritis illustrate the variety of arthritis, highlighting the significance of a comprehensive diagnosis to develop appropriate treatment programs for afflicted people. While some types of arthritis have similar symptoms, knowing which kind you have is critical for adopting focused therapies.

## Arthritis Common Symptoms

Arthritis causes a variety of symptoms, the intensity and mix of which varies greatly across people. Joint discomfort, edema, stiffness, and a limited range of motion are common symptoms. Arthritic pain is often characterized as aching, throbbing, or stabbing, and it may be more severe after periods of inactivity or heavy usage of the afflicted joint.

Swelling is another common symptom caused by inflammation

of the joint lining. This might result in a noticeably larger joint and add to the sensation of stiffness. Stiffness is a common symptom of arthritis, especially in the mornings or after extended periods of rest. Individuals suffering from arthritis may find it difficult to commence movement, but the stiffness usually decreases with modest, steady exercise.

Another effect of arthritis is a reduced range of motion. Individuals may find it more difficult to do common actions that involve joint mobility, such as walking, climbing stairs, or gripping things, as joint flexibility declines. The effect of arthritis on movement may have a substantial influence on a person's freedom and general well-being.

Fatigue is a symptom that is not limited to the damaged joints but is present in many people with arthritis. Chronic pain and inflammation linked with the illness may cause persistent weariness, interfering with everyday tasks and contributing to a general feeling of malaise.

Individuals with various types of arthritis, such as rheumatoid arthritis, may also have systemic symptoms. Fever, weight loss, and overall sensations of ill-health are examples. Such systemic symptoms signal that the inflammatory process has spread beyond the joints and has begun to damage other regions of the body.

It's crucial to understand that arthritic symptoms may change over time, with flare-ups marked by greater symptoms and remissions characterized by symptoms that may lessen or become more bearable. Because arthritis is unpredictable, it emphasizes the significance of continual medical care and tailored treatment regimens.

Arthritis is a complicated and varied set of diseases that affect millions of individuals throughout the globe. Understanding its nature, varied forms, and prevalent symptoms is critical for successful care and increased quality of life for individuals afflicted. Each kind of arthritis demands a unique therapeutic strategy, from the wear and tear of osteoarthritis to the immunological reaction in rheumatoid arthritis.

As medical research progresses, so does our knowledge of arthritis and the development of new therapies. Early diagnosis and management are critical to properly treating arthritis and minimizing its effects on joints, general health, and everyday activities. We can better help people living with arthritis and try to improve their quality of life by promoting awareness and cultivating a full knowledge of the illness.

# CHAPTER TWO

## Arthritis Diagnosis Techniques: From Early Detection to Diagnosis

Early identification of arthritis is critical for initiating timely therapies and successfully treating the illness. However, arthritis refers to a group of diseases, each with its own set of symptoms and diagnostic problems. Osteoarthritis, rheumatoid arthritis, gout, and psoriatic arthritis are all common kinds of arthritis.

## Clinical Examination

A comprehensive clinical examination is often used by medical professionals to begin the diagnosis procedure. This includes a thorough review of the patient's medical history, a physical examination, and an evaluation of symptoms. Typical signs that healthcare practitioners check for during this examination include joint discomfort, stiffness, edema, and reduced range of motion.

## Imaging Investigations

Imaging investigations are usually used to gain a better look at the joints and discover any abnormalities. X-rays, magnetic resonance imaging (MRI), and ultrasound may aid in the visualization of joint structures, the detection of inflammation, and the assessment of joint damage.

## Blood Tests

Blood tests are very useful in the diagnosis of inflammatory arthritis, such as rheumatoid arthritis. C-reactive protein (CRP) and erythrocyte sedimentation rate (ESR) values that are elevated might suggest inflammation in the body.

# Arthrocentesis (Joint Aspiration)

If the diagnosis is still ambiguous, joint aspiration may be done. A tiny sample of synovial fluid from the afflicted joint is taken for examination. Crystals, inflammatory cells, or infection may all give useful diagnostic information.

# CHAPTER THREE

## Genetic Testing

Some types of arthritis, such as ankylosing spondylitis and psoriatic arthritis, are inherited. Genetic testing may assist in the identification of particular markers linked with various disorders, allowing for a more precise diagnosis.

## Traditional Arthritis Treatments

When a diagnosis of arthritis is made, healthcare practitioners often seek standard treatment options to control symptoms and enhance the patient's quality of life.

• Nonsteroidal Anti-Inflammatory Drugs (NSAIDs): These treatments assist in decreasing inflammation and discomfort. Ibuprofen and naproxen are two common NSAIDs.

• Disease-Modifying Antirheumatic Drugs (DMARDs): DMARDs are used to delay the course of inflammatory arthritis, such as rheumatoid arthritis.

• Corticosteroids: Because of their significant anti-inflammatory properties, corticosteroids may be recommended in situations of severe inflammation.

• Physical therapists play an important role in assisting arthritis patients in maintaining joint function and reducing pain. Stretching and targeted workouts may enhance mobility and strengthen supporting muscles.

3. Occupational Therapy: • Occupational therapists work with patients to improve their capacity to conduct everyday tasks. They propose adaptive tactics and assistive technology to make everyday activities easier to handle.

• Intra-articular injections of corticosteroids or hyaluronic acid may be delivered directly into afflicted joints to offer regional pain and inflammation alleviation.

## Pain Management Techniques

Pain management is an important element of arthritis therapy, and a multifaceted strategy is often required to produce the best outcomes.

1. Hot and Cold Therapies: Applying heat or cold to damaged joints may help relieve pain and inflammation. Warm compresses or heating pads help relieve tight

joints, and cold packs can relieve acute inflammation.

• TENS treatment includes the use of a tiny, battery-powered device that delivers moderate electrical shocks to nerve endings, disrupting pain signals and delivering relief.

• Practices such as meditation, deep breathing, and guided imagery may help manage pain by increasing relaxation and lowering stress, which frequently exacerbates arthritic symptoms.

• Acupuncture involves the insertion of tiny needles into particular spots on the body. Many people with arthritis report less pain and better joint function following acupuncture treatments.

## Diet and Nutrition in the Treatment of Arthritis

Diet and nutrition are important in controlling arthritis symptoms and improving overall joint health. While there is no treatment for arthritis, some dietary choices may help decrease inflammation and enhance joint function.

1. Anti-Inflammatory Foods: Including anti-inflammatory foods in your diet might be useful. Fatty fish (high in omega-3 fatty acids),

nuts, seeds, fruits, vegetables, and whole grains are examples.

2. Omega-3 Fatty Acids: • Taking fish oil supplements or eating fatty fish like salmon and mackerel may supply omega-3 fatty acids, which have anti-inflammatory properties.

3. Turmeric and Ginger: Turmeric and ginger are both anti-inflammatory. Incorporating these spices into dishes or drinking them as teas might help relieve arthritic symptoms.

# CHAPTER FOUR

## Maintaining a Healthy Weight

Excess body weight may place additional strain on joints, especially in weight-bearing regions. A balanced diet and maintaining a healthy weight may help lessen the strain on arthritic joints.

Finally, arthritis diagnosis entails a mix of clinical examination, imaging investigations, and laboratory testing. Traditional treatments, such as drugs and therapies, try to alleviate symptoms while also improving joint function. Pain treatment techniques take a comprehensive approach, with food and nutrition playing an important part in total joint health. A holistic approach to arthritis care takes into account each individual's unique symptoms and demands, enabling a higher quality of life for people suffering from this difficult illness.

Individuals dealing with issues such as arthritis frequently find consolation and progress via a diverse strategy that combines physical therapy, exercise, novel medical techniques, and complementary and alternative therapies. We go into the junction of these factors in this thorough investigation, stressing their significance in improving joint health, controlling arthritis, and creating a holistic approach to well-being.

## Exercise and Physical Therapy for Joint Health

Physical therapy is critical in treating joint health, especially for those suffering from arthritis. Physical therapy's main objective is to increase mobility, decrease discomfort, and improve general functioning.

A good physical therapist tailors exercises to each patient's demands and limits, promoting a tailored approach.

Physical rehabilitation programs must include joint-friendly activities. These exercises are designed to improve flexibility, strength, and endurance without putting excessive strain on the joints. Low-impact activities such as swimming, walking, and cycling are often suggested for arthritis patients to preserve joint health and avoid additional damage. These activities not only help with arthritic symptoms but also improve general cardiovascular fitness.

Range-of-motion exercises, in addition to standard exercises, are regularly added to physical therapy regimens. These exercises are designed to maintain or increase joint flexibility, as well as to avoid stiffness and promote optimum joint function. Exercises that concentrate on the muscles around the afflicted joints give extra support, reducing stress on the joints themselves.

## Innovative Medical Approaches to Arthritis

Medical science advancements have opened the path for novel methods of arthritis management. Biologic medicines are one such significant discovery. Biologics target particular immune system components that cause inflammation, which is a major contributor to arthritis. These medications may successfully decrease joint inflammation and limit the course of some kinds of arthritis by modifying the immune response.

Furthermore, regenerative medicine has promise in the treatment of arthritis. Stem cell treatment is a kind of regenerative medicine, that uses a patient's stem cells to heal damaged tissues and decrease joint inflammation. While research is still in its early phases, the potential for stem cell therapy to change arthritis treatment provides a ray of hope for people looking for alternatives to traditional techniques.

Another notable improvement in arthritis care is precision medicine. This method personalizes treatment regimens based on a person's genetic makeup, allowing for more focused and successful treatments. Healthcare practitioners may enhance treatment options and improve results by identifying the unique genetic components that contribute to an individual's arthritis.

# The Mind-Body Connection: Arthritis and Mental Health

The mind-body link is critical in arthritis management. Chronic pain and physical restrictions associated with arthritis may have a substantial psychological influence on an individual's mental health.

Depression and anxiety are widespread among arthritis patients, underscoring the need for a comprehensive approach to management.

Mindfulness-based techniques like meditation and yoga have shown potential in improving mental health in people with arthritis. These techniques stress being present at the moment and maintaining a positive mentality, which may be especially helpful in dealing with the emotional toll of chronic pain.

Cognitive-behavioral therapy (CBT) is another effective treatment for the mental health effects of arthritis. CBT assists people in re-framing negative thinking patterns, developing pain-coping techniques, and improving general emotional resilience.

# CHAPTER FIVE

# Alternative and complementary therapies

Alternative and complementary treatments provide extra options for controlling arthritic symptoms and increasing general well-being.

Acupuncture, an ancient Chinese treatment that involves inserting small needles into particular places on the body, has gained popularity for its ability to relieve arthritic pain. While the processes behind acupuncture's efficacy are still being researched, many people experience alleviation from joint discomfort and greater mobility.

Dietary supplements, such as omega-3 fatty acids and glucosamine, are often investigated as adjunctive treatments for arthritis.

Fish oil contains omega-3 fatty acids, which have anti-inflammatory qualities and may help relieve joint pain and stiffness. Glucosamine, a naturally occurring component in cartilage, is often used as a supplement to improve joint health and perhaps decrease the course of arthritis.

Herbal medicines, such as turmeric and ginger, are also popular for their anti-inflammatory qualities. Curcumin, a chemical found in turmeric, is renowned for its ability to decrease inflammation and improve arthritic symptoms.

While additional study is required to completely understand the effectiveness of these complementary treatments, many people find them useful as part of a comprehensive strategy for arthritis care.

Finally, managing joint health, particularly in the setting of arthritis, requires a holistic and integrated approach. Physical therapy and focused exercises provide the groundwork for preserving joint functioning, while cutting-edge medical techniques such as biologics and regenerative medicine provide cutting-edge treatments.

It is critical to recognize the mind-body link and treat mental health via methods such as mindfulness and cognitive-behavioral therapy. Complementary and alternative treatments, such as acupuncture and nutritional supplements, flesh out the holistic approach, giving people a wide arsenal for controlling arthritis and promoting overall well-being. As the healthcare environment evolves, taking a multidimensional approach to joint health is critical for improving the quality of life for persons living with arthritis.

## Arthritis Wellness Lifestyle Modifications

Arthritis is a chronic disorder characterized by joint inflammation, which causes pain, stiffness, and decreased mobility. While there is no treatment for arthritis, some lifestyle changes may considerably help general well-being and symptom relief for people who suffer from it. These changes take a comprehensive approach, including physical activity, diet, stress management, and other aspects that affect the quality of life of people with arthritis.

## Examples of Case Studies: Arthritis Patients' Real-Life Experiences

Real-life case studies provide solid evidence of how lifestyle changes may make a significant impact on arthritis management. Sarah, a 45-year-old woman with rheumatoid arthritis, is one such example. Sarah initially struggled with everyday tasks and had constant joint discomfort. She saw a considerable improvement in her joint flexibility and discomfort after including frequent low-impact workouts like swimming and eating an anti-inflammatory diet rich in omega-3 fatty acids.

James, a 60-year-old man with knee osteoarthritis, is another inspirational story. Rather than relying only on medicine, James integrated weight management into his regimen, dropping extra pounds to relieve stress on his joints. In addition, he followed his physical therapist's recommendations for strength training activities, which not only provided muscular support around his knees but also improved his entire well-being.

These case studies show that each person's road to arthritis relief is unique, necessitating a customized strategy that incorporates numerous lifestyle adjustments adapted to particular circumstances.

# CHAPTER SIX

# Practical Arthritis Tips for Everyday Life

1. Consistent Exercise: Regular low-impact exercise is essential for preserving joint flexibility and decreasing stiffness. Swimming, walking, and mild yoga are all good activities. To establish an appropriate workout plan, it is important to speak with a healthcare expert or a physical therapist.

2. Nutritional Balance: Adopting an anti-inflammatory diet will help manage arthritis symptoms. Anti-inflammatory foods include

fatty fish and flaxseeds, which are high in omega-3 fatty acids. Including a mix of fruits, vegetables, and whole grains in your diet will help you acquire the nutrients you need to support your overall joint health.

3. Weight Control: Maintaining a healthy weight is particularly essential for those with arthritis since excess weight puts extra strain on the joints. Implementing a healthy diet and regular exercise may help with weight control and, as a result, decrease arthritic symptoms.

4. Joint Protection strategies: Using joint protection strategies in everyday activities may help reduce stress on damaged joints. Simple measures such as employing assistive devices, and ergonomic equipment, and adopting good body mechanics may help to preserve joint function.

5. Stress Reduction: Chronic stress may aggravate arthritis symptoms. Stress management practices including meditation, deep breathing exercises, and mindfulness may help decrease stress and improve general well-being.

6. Adequate Rest and Sleep: People with arthritis must have enough rest and sleep. Creating a pleasant sleep environment, sticking to a regular sleep schedule, and practicing relaxation methods may all help you sleep better and manage your symptoms better.

7. periodic Health Check-ups: It is important to evaluate arthritis symptoms regularly and to schedule periodic check-ups with healthcare specialists. This enables fast changes to treatment regimens and guarantees that any new difficulties are addressed as soon as possible.

8. Participation in a Supportive Community: Joining support groups or connecting with a community of people experiencing similar issues may give emotional support and useful insights. Sharing experiences and learning from others may help people feel more connected and empowered.

## Conclusion

Finally, controlling arthritis requires a diversified strategy that goes beyond medicinal measures. Lifestyle changes, as shown by real-life case studies and practical recommendations, play a critical role in improving the overall well-being of people with arthritis.

These changes include components of physical activity, diet, stress management, and other factors, underlining the significance of a comprehensive approach to arthritis treatment.

Each person's path to arthritis relief is unique, and finding the appropriate mix of lifestyle changes takes time and perseverance. Individuals may improve their joint health, reduce discomfort, and improve their overall quality of life by integrating these practical recommendations into their everyday lives. With continuous research and a greater knowledge of arthritis, there is optimism for additional breakthroughs in lifestyle-based methods for treating this chronic illness.